Live
SUCCESSFULLY!

BOOK No. 4

MEMORY,
CONCENTRATION AND HABIT

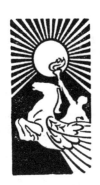

TRY THESE TESTS!

After you have read Book No. 4, entitled "MEMORY, CONCENTRATION AND HABIT" you will find it helpful to ask yourself these questions. The answers will be found inside. Do not break the seal before you have written out or decided your answers. Questions 7, 8, 9 and 10 are general intelligence tests and the rest of the questions are based on the book.

1 Suppose you are playing the game of remembering a number of objects on the table. Here is an alphabetical list of things displayed :—candle, cigarette card, envelope, gold watch, match-box, newspaper, pencil, penknife, penny, photograph, ruler, sealing wax, sovereign. Suggest how you could link them in an order which would be easily remembered.

2 How many of the objects below can you memorise in one minute ? Time yourself by the clock, then write down a list of as many as you can remember.

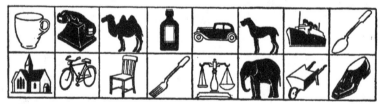

3 To test your powers of concentration, see how long you need to read the following before you discover the one item that is missing in each :—

(a) RLQNFKHCIDUXMOGBAEZYWPJTV ;
(b) 763908251 ;
(c) April, November, August, February, September, June, December, July, October, January, May ;
(d) Saturday, Wednesday, Monday, Thursday, Tuesday, Sunday.

ANSWERS

TO TEST

1 The *gold watch* suggests the gold *sovereign*, which in a different sense means the same as *ruler*, which reminds us of the *pencil*, which is sharpened with the *penknife*, which will open the *envelope*, which suggests the *sealing wax*, which suggests the *candle* and thus the *match-box*, which reminds us of cigarettes and the *cigarette card*, which suggests the *photograph*, which brings us to the *newspaper*, which may be bought with the *penny*.

2 Few people could memorise the objects in one minute and those who succeed in memorising twelve or more have every reason to feel satisfied with their memory.

3 The missing items are :
(a) S ; (b) 4 ; (c) March ; (d) Friday.
In the case of (b) and (d) a quick person would arrive at the answer in 2 seconds, while the average time would probably be 3 seconds. In the case of (c) the two times would be 3 and 4 seconds respectively, and in the case of (a) they would be 15 and 20 seconds.

QUESTIONS

4 (a) 34 is the double of 17; (b) the reverse of the famous date 1066; (c) exactly 1000 years after the outbreak of the Great War; (d) one dozen followed by three dozen. Alternatively $1 \times 2 \times 3 = 6$.

5 Memory always works better when it is allied to natural interest. Learning tables for their own sake will strike a child as useless and uninteresting.

6 (a) to the right of the observer; (b) blue; (c) yellow and black; (d) blue; (e) the Bank of England; (f) a lion.

7 As she heard correctly that the third letter was E, she had no need to ask for what it stood.

8 The inverted book indicates that it has been moved and hurriedly replaced. The document is probably inside the book.

9 The other hairdresser was the son's mother.

10 Because the key will fall into the locked letter-box.

4 Suggest an easy way of remembering the following telephone numbers :—
(a) 1734 ; (b) 6601 ; (c) 2914 ; (d) 1236.

5 Explain why a young boy or girl learns to reckon money and the giving of change quickly while playing a shop, but is often rather slow in learning money tables at school.

6 Try to answer the following questions by picturing the objects in your mind :—
(a) Which way does Britannia face on a penny ?
(b) What colour is a 2½d. stamp ?
(c) What colour is an A.A. road-sign ?
(d) What colour is the outside ring of the markings on the wings of an R.A.F. plane ?
(e) What is the picture on the back of a pound note ?
(f) What animal is shown at the beginning of every Metro-Goldwyn-Mayer film ?

7 What remark in this telephone talk suggests that the speaker is not very intelligent or at least weak in concentration ?
" No, she is not at home, sir. Whom shall I say rang ? . . . I did not catch the name, sir, will you please spell it ? . . . G for goat, R for rose. . . . Yes, I got that. E for what, sir ? . . . Empty. Right, I'll remember. And G for goat, sir. Thank you, Mr. Greg."

8 A thief has been disturbed while endeavouring to escape with a valuable document. He has hurriedly secreted it some-where. Can you discover a clue in the scene illustrated on the right ?

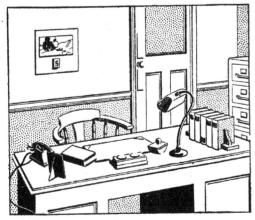

9 " Two hairdressers glanced at us through the window of their establishment. Later we were not particularly surprised to learn that one of them was the father of the other hair-dresser's son." How can this be explained ?

10 The professor on holiday telephoned to his secretary :
" Why are you not forwarding my letters ? " he asked.
" You forgot to leave me the key of your letter-box," she said.
" How silly of me ! I shall send it at once," he replied, and he hung up the receiver and summoned a page boy for an envelope and stamp.
Why is it likely that he still will not get his letters ?

CONTENTS
OF BOOK No. 4

WHAT
MENTAL EFFICIENCY
MEANS TO YOU

THE human mind is a marvellous instrument. It provides us all with miraculous powers. But like other sensitive mechanisms, it needs constant attention if it is to work at its best.

You have seen in Books 2 and 3 how to deal with the maladjustments of inferiority feeling and fear which may handicap the mind at times. Now we come naturally to the inspiring subject of mental efficiency—how to remember, how to concentrate, how to get the best possible performance from the wonderful mental instrument with which you are endowed.

That is the subject of this Book. To a large extent it is a " key " Book in the Plan. All twelve volumes are important, but the lessons this one teaches are *imperative*.

In all walks of life, in all our work and all our play, a certain average level of mental efficiency is necessary. We need mention only briefly here how you use memory and concentration every day, how your habits are best if under *your* control instead of their controlling you, how your will-power and imagination both affect you daily.

But how much more important are these qualities when you are engaged on the development of success and happiness through a definite and painstaking Plan !

You will want to concentrate on this and every other Book to get the greatest possible value from them. You will want to make certain that your powers of memory are such that you can retain and use the lessons you learn.

Habits of happiness and industry you will certainly desire to develop. They are vital to keep your interest at that height which makes self-development an adventure rather than a task. Then with imagination to show you how to use what you learn, and will-power to maintain your enthusiasm, how can anything stop you on the road to success and happiness ?

Do you wonder we say this is one of the " key " Books ? Let us get on, then, and see how mental efficiency may be mastered !

1. HOW HABIT CAN HELP YOU

VERY often, when people are taken to task for slovenly and careless behaviour, they excuse themselves by saying that they have formed a "habit" which they cannot break. We heard of habitual criminals; of a person being habitually lazy, and so on. It almost is as if, once a person has formed undesirable habits, he is irreparably lost—but this is not so, as we shall presently learn.

Later, we shall see how habits are essential to an ordered, systematic life—how they should become the servants of the individual—part of a harmonious personality. It is when his personality has as its foundation *bad* habits, that the individual becomes "out of tune" with society and himself.

WHAT HABITS ARE

First, let us examine what is meant by the term habit; then we can consider the next problem—the part habit plays in your daily life. In everyday language, you may use the phrase " getting into a habit " in very much the same way as you sometimes speak of people " getting into a groove." In psychological language, if you perform an action once, certain nervous and mental lines of communication are developed.

The first time you do anything, the mental process involves a decision, a delay while the necessary adjustments are made, as between mind and body. Just as the first time a key is turned in a lock, the mechanism is stiff, and hard to operate.

The second time you perform the same action the paths operating backwards and forwards between nerves and muscles are already in existence to some extent, and so the delay is less. After constant repetition, no delay at all ensues. You perform the action without any mental effort at all, and often without even being aware of what you are doing.

HOW HABITS DEVELOP

If you wish to study how a habit is developed, try this experiment. Take a mirror, and place it upright on a table. With a ruler, draw a six-pointed star on a sheet of paper. Put the sheet of paper flat on the table in front of the mirror, then, with a pencil, and guided only by the reflected image, try to trace around the star. The first time this will be difficult, because movement is in a reverse direction to normal. Then, trace around the star again. Each time you repeat the new movement, it will become

IT HAS BEEN SUGGESTED THAT WE⌉
⌈MORE READ TO ABLE BE SHOULD⌋
⌊QUICKLY IF WE STARTED FROM ONE⌉
⌈READ THEN AND LINE THE OF END⌋
⌊BACK ALONG THE OTHER FROM⌉
⌈HABIT A IS IT BUT.LEFT TO RIGHT⌋
⌊WHICH NEEDS A FEW LINES OF⌉
⌈TO USED GET WE BEFORE READING⌋
⌊IT AS YOU WILL HAVE REALISED !

HOW A HABIT DEVELOPS

The curious idea of speeding up reading by starting from the end of the line where the previous line ends (instead of making a leap with the eye back to the left of the page as we do now) can easily be grasped with practice. Habit makes it easy after the first few lines. Read this out once or twice and see how you speed up with practice.

easier, because the muscles in your hand become accustomed to acting in a new way. They acquire, in fact, a new habit.

A familiar example of habit forming is seen in a person learning to drive a motor-car. At first hands, feet, eyes and brain work separately. The learner concentrates on gear-changing, perhaps, and forgets to watch the road. But with practice the various movements needed become almost automatic, and can be performed together without effort. The learner has acquired the habit of driving.

When we are born, we have our lives before us in which to form good or bad habits. Once formed, a bad habit is difficult to eradicate ; but good habits are the foundation for a full and useful life. Habits formed in childhood nearly always persist, right through life. Habits of cleanliness, tidiness, method, perseverance, concentration, clear thinking, if cultivated during your early life, persist as invaluable assets when you reach more mature years.

WITHOUT HABITS, OUR MINDS WOULD BE INTOLERABLY OVERWORKED

William James, the psychologist, in his " Principles of Psychology," has asked the question : " What would happen if every time you dressed, you had to stop and consider what to do next ? " The answer is easy. Instead of taking half an hour, or less, it would take you perhaps five or six times as long, because each time you wanted to put on anything, you would have to decide whether you should lift the right or the left leg first, put your arm into the right or the left sleeve, brush your hair before you put on your collar or blouse, and so on.

Life in such circumstances would become intolerable. You would be so busy deciding what to do next that ultimately you would do very little—and probably even that little, unsatisfactorily. Instead of leaving details such as waking up at a certain hour, dressing, breakfasting, catching a train, or the minor routine of your work to habit, and reserving the greater part of your mental energy for decisions that matter, your mind would become so overworked by the necessity for decision on detail, that you would never progress. Develop good habits to take care of the details of your life, then your mind will be fresher and freer to grapple with the real problems confronting you.

SET OUT TO CONTROL YOUR HABITS

Good habits, properly controlled and developed, are valuable assets ; bad habits are a sign of mental weakness, poor self-training, and result in disorganised living. Once formed, habits are difficult to break, regardless of whether they are good or bad.

Suppose, that every week-day for a month, or longer, circumstances have forced you to reach your office at eight o'clock in the morning. At the end of this period, you will have formed the habit of doing this. Automatically, you rise early. If, suddenly, it only becomes necessary for you to be there at nine o'clock, you will find yourself tending to arrive before time. Taking this a step further, the reverse also holds good. The more frequently you arrive late at the office, the harder it will become to arrive on time.

The fundamental principle is that the more often you do the wrong thing, the easier it will become to do it again. The more frequently you discipline yourself to act as you should, the more automatic, the easier, this will be. Once you discover you are developing a bad habit, the sooner you train yourself to act differently, the less effort you will have to make in breaking the bad habit.

IF HABITS ARE NOT CONTROLLED, THEY WILL CONTROL YOU

To break a habit requires concentration and mental effort. For example, you may form the habit of crossing a certain field on your way to the railway station. Then, one day, a fence is put up to block the path. The first few days after you have discovered you can no longer go that way, it requires mental concentration to go by another route. Then, one morning, you are thinking about other matters ; suddenly, you find yourself automatically going towards the field you have formed the habit of crossing. Your habit has taken charge of you, once your concentration has been relaxed.

If you merely let yourself drift, without mental effort to control the direction you take, you will form habits which will carry you along a path of least resistance. Then, unless you subject yourself to severe self-discipline, you will drift still further, from bad to worse. If you had been careful to develop the right habits in the first place, although this might have required more effort, subsequently, life would have proceeded smoothly, and been better regulated. *Remember, it is easier to form a good habit than to break a bad one.*

HOW HABITS CAN BE CONTROLLED

Before setting forth on any course of action, decide whether it is the right one. Then pursue it fearlessly. By repetition, reduce it to a habit so that the need for mental effort, when you are again called upon to act similarly, will not arise. You will act efficiently, without mental effort ; your mind will be free to utilise its energy in concentrating upon other important decisions.

If, later on, events show that your course of action is not the best one, do not hesitate to change. Discipline yourself to create a habit involving a more satisfactory course of action.

Concentrate, until the new habit has become established in the place of the old one ; until it has become mechanical, and there is no danger that, when something else is uppermost in your mind, you will automatically drift back to the old habit. *Make habit your servant, not your master.*

REPLACE BAD HABITS WITH GOOD NEW ONES

The controlling, or repressing, of bad habits is difficult—especially if they are deep seated in your mental make-up by reason of frequent repetition over a long period of time. Just as the mountain stream that has cut its way deep into the rocks is hard to stem, or divert to another channel, so an established habit cannot be repressed, or changed to a new one, without mental disturbance.

Make a list of your habits, decide which tend to hinder your progress. It may be that you have become accustomed to mental inertia in certain directions, that you have acquired an aversion to physical effort, or that you have found it easier to be careless in your work, your appearance, your manner of speaking. Perhaps, for instance, you do not answer letters promptly, or are not careful to clean your shoes every morning.

Failures in these matters have become habits without you being aware of it. It is not sufficient to realise these bad habits are a hindrance to you. You must go further. You must first of all repress them, and then set to work to learn new and better habits built up on a sound foundation of self-control.

UPROOTING A HABIT LEAVES A GAP

You have read of active business men retiring and then pining for their work, at a complete loss what to do. This is because they have cultivated a habit of being active in their business. When they retire, circumstances require them to be less active. The formation of a habit represents the creation of a channel for the expression of energy in a definite way. If this is blocked, and the energy cannot find another outlet, mental conflict, unhappiness, and discontent result.

If you have formed a habit, do not imagine it can be repressed ruthlessly without serious effects. The business man, when he retires, and if he is wise, will find an outlet for his energy, by playing golf, by acquiring other interests; and the chain-smoker who gives up cigarettes may profitably satisfy himself with sweets. That is, one should deliberately create new habits to replace the old ones.

When you are trying to form a habit which seems to you desirable but difficult to cultivate, it is good to provide yourself with a strong motive for doing as you intend. The following story shows how an incentive can be provided —though few readers will be prepared to repeat the exact details of the experience !

FORMING A HABIT

It is told of Simeon, the famous vicar of Holy Trinity, Cambridge, that he found it extremely difficult to get up in the morning. In desperation he decided to take drastic steps to attain the habit of early rising. He promised himself he would give half a crown to his bedmaker on any occasion when he did not rise at the appointed time.

On the morning following when it was time to get up he found a very sound reason for staying in bed. He argued that his bedmaker needed the half a crown more than he did !

But when at last he was really awake, he resolved the next time he missed he would throw a guinea into the Cam. Next day he was poorer by that guinea. But, as he records, richer in that he had made a step towards acquiring the desired habit.

When a habit is in the earlier stages of being cultivated consciously, either as a new form of activity, or to replace another old one, there will come to you temptations to revert to old methods. You may persuade yourself that just one exception will not matter very much. This is a most dangerous period. To permit a single exception will undo much of what you have achieved. The agreement between mind and body, that you have sought to make automatic, will be disturbed. You may even have to begin all over again.

The effort then necessary to revert once more to the new habit will be considerable. It will seem easier to go on and make more exceptions, and so you will begin to drift again. School yourself against temptations to make exceptions to a habit you are seeking to establish. You will obtain the ultimate result you desire much sooner and with less total effort. It will require self-discipline, but, in the end, what you achieve will be worth while.

THIS CHAPTER HAS TOLD YOU

1. Habits make life automatically easier. Without them, our minds would be intolerably overworked. They make it possible to act as we have done before, but without further mental effort.

2. *See how a habit is developed by the exercise with a mirror on page 8.*

3. *Habits are difficult to break. But it is worth making an extra effort, because if you do not control your habits, they will control you.*

4. *Be careful to lay down good sound habits. A little effort in the beginning saves much trouble later.*

5. *Changing habits is difficult. It is not sufficient just to weed out the old habit. That leaves a gap that will make you unhappy until it is filled.*

6. *Create new habits to replace the old. Self-control and concentration are essential. Permit no exceptions to the new habit and eventually it will gain the firm grip you desire.*

2. HOW TO USE IMAGINATION

EVERY experience, however unimportant, in some way modifies your mental structure so that recollections or mental pictures of these experiences may arise in your mind long afterwards. It is impossible to form a mental picture of anything you have never experienced. If you lose your eyesight, you may form visual images of scenes you have visited long ago but, if you have been born blind, you will never be able to have a mental vision. Your mind is always active recalling experiences, and adding to them elements from other experiences. This process is known as imagination or phantasy.

IMAGINATION'S MANY FORMS

People differ in imagination : some are said to have vivid imaginations, others none at all. The painter, recreating a new whole composed of a number of elements from his experience, is giving practical expression to a recombination of what he has seen. The novelist reshuffles his experience ; his stories are combinations of his own experiences, or of experiences he has found in books or learned in conversation with others. The skill, or the degree of novelty, with which the painter or novelist makes these new combinations shows the creative quality of his imagination.

When you recall an experience you may do so in various ways. Suppose you recollect your first visit to a friend's house. You may form mental images of what the garden looked like, how the house was furnished, and so on. These are visual images. Recollection of the scent of the flowers—*smell images*—may come to you ; or the soft feeling as you trod on the grass— *tactile, or touch images ;* or the noise of the traffic in the street—*auditory images ;* or the muscular effort involved in climbing up the stairs— *motile or movement images.* You will learn more about these different kinds of memory on page 50 and the succeeding pages.

The most common type, and the one which predominates with most people, is the *visual image,* although the other types are experienced by the majority of individuals at different times. If a person recalls images based on past experience to any extent, and especially if he recombines the various elements to produce a novel result, he is said to have a vivid imagination.

DREAMS, PHANTASIES, WISHES, THOUGHTS

You have had many moments in your life when your mind has formed and reformed

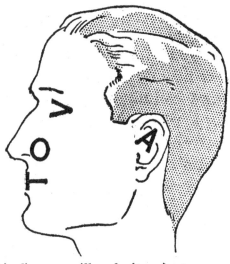

This diagram will make it easier to remember the different senses and the way they help us in memorising. V stands for Visual (sight); O for Odile (smell); T for Tactile (touch and taste); A for Auditory (hearing)

images from the past. If this is done extensively during your waking hours, you will be called a day-dreamer. At night, when your body is resting, and you are asleep, past experiences flood back into your recollection. The elements may be combined simply, or fantastically distorted, in what are known as dreams.

Psychologists explain dreams partly by saying that they fulfil what we wish for. The poor man dreams of possessing riches; the child, of the toys his parents cannot afford to buy for him; the individual who, in real life, lacks the energy to achieve his ambition, dreams that he has done so. Thus, when you cannot get what you want in reality, you may seek satisfaction in dreams ; you give the various elements in your mind a new direction, when you dream, until they are combined into the picture you want—with yourself in the centre.

If you do so consciously during waking hours, with a definite object in view, the result will be something new and useful. You are making proper use of your imagination.

But if you allow yourself to create a dream picture simply because real life has denied what you desire, then you begin to live falsely. You are in danger of finding so much satisfaction in your dream world that you become entirely divorced from the responsibilities of your real existence. You come to live in a world created by your imagination.

DIRECT YOUR IMAGINATION

On the other hand, if you create a mental picture of what you would like to be, consciously strive to achieve it, and direct all your energies towards doing so, then you will reach your goal or, if you do not, at least you will know the satisfaction of having tried.

If you have never seriously thought how you use imagination yourself, think about it now.

Pull yourself up and ask the question :

" What kind of force is imagination in my life ? Is it a spur sending me onwards ? Is it a great creative force in my life ? Is it harnessed so that it leads to practical achievement, or is it my foe ? Do I use imagination in morbid and uncreative ways ? Do I spend my time thinking about things which may never happen to me ? Do I use imagination in small and petty ways and never rise to the heights ?"

You must be frank with yourself. Imagination, in any case, is a powerful factor. If only you learn to use it in the right way you will find that life becomes a different affair. It will be more adventurous, it will be more worthwhile, and it is certain in the truest sense that it will be more successful.

WHERE NEW IDEAS COME FROM

You have probably seen many new inventions that have made fortunes for those who had the imagination to think of them, and the energy to apply what they originally evolved as a mental image. Many brilliant inventors have failed to reap the benefit of their work because they have been dreamers only, and have not been able to make practical use of their creations. *Success demands concrete application of what you have built up in your imagination.*

Often, when a new idea has been explained,

you have asked yourself why you did not think of it. The reason may not be that you have not had the essential experience or training. More probably it is because your imagination has not been so trained that you are able to re-combine the elements of your experience in the form necessary to produce the result that has surprised you with its simplicity—once you have seen how it has been done. New ideas are very often nothing more than a rearrangement of old experiences—possibly a complete reshuffle of elements, or perhaps only a minor addition to an existing combination.

It was because men with imagination saw birds flying in the air, that they imagined they, too, could fly. If the situation had remained thus, without any effort being made to fulfil this dream, nothing would have been achieved. It was because energy, experience and scientific knowledge were brought to bear, to give practical expression to a dream, that aeroplanes have developed.

IMAGINATION MAY MISLEAD

On the other hand, not every goal imagination presents is capable of attainment. Because you are deeply interested in films and love to picture yourself as a successful actor, it does not follow that you are therefore fitted for a film career. Imagination, to be a useful driving force, must be harnessed by the powers and abilities you really do possess.

Great talkers are seldom great doers. Think, then act. Do not spend your time talking about what you are going to do, because then the chances are that all your energy will be expended in chatter. Invariably, the person who describes at length what he is going to do, is merely another type of day-dreamer. Instead of obtaining satisfaction by *doing*, he obtains all the satisfaction he desires from telling people what he intends to do.

The man who achieves his goal rarely discusses his actions at length with anyone, unless he has a definite purpose in doing so. He proceeds with calm, silent confidence. He *thinks* instead of talking. The irresponsible person chatters to all and sundry of how he is going to succeed, and how he proposes to go about it.

DON'T FORGET TO ACT

Let your imagination set the goal for you. This will provide the incentive. Imagine yourself having achieved your object. Picture the advantages, the satisfaction you will enjoy. Without such a stimulus, your efforts will lack the dynamic force necessary to sustain and bring them to a successful conclusion. But don't forget that you must *act* in addition to dreaming about acting. Control your imagination, so that all the powers within you are directed towards giving concrete expression to your ambitious dreams. Then you must succeed. Nothing will hold you back.

**EXERCISES IN CREATIVE IMAGINATION :
THINGS TO DO**

1. The most self-revealing test of all is to make a list of the ambitions you have dreamt of achieving during, say, the last five years. Note against each what positive action you have taken. If the list is a long one, you must learn to control your imagination. If there are many instances where you have taken no action, you must train yourself to dream less and act more.

2. As a beginning in the training of your imagination, take anything you have done during the day. Think about it. Consider every factor involved. Turn over in your mind how you did it ; the difficulties you had ; how you have seen other people do it. If necessary, consult books about how it should be done. Recombine all these ideas ; bring your imagination to bear in an effort to evolve a new procedure. When you have succeeded in doing

this, think about what the effects will be if you apply the method you have worked out. Then, to-morrow—act. Put your new idea into operation.

THIS CHAPTER HAS TOLD YOU

1. The mind is always recalling experiences and adding to them elements from other experiences. That is how imagination works.

2. Imagination takes many forms : dreams, phantasy, wishful thinking, creative planning, and so on.

3. We should not allow imaginative excursions to take the place of action. Imagination should be a spur to action.

4. A far-seeing imagination combined with a practical outlook will produce the most fruitful ideas. Dreams may hold a fortune—but not unless they can stand the test of practice.

5. Imagination is dangerous unless focused on concrete objectives. Do not allow talk to replace action when you are imagining some aim.

6. Picture the goal as already achieved. In this way imagination will " raise steam " to drive you forward.

3. THE WAY TO INCREASE WILL-POWER

Y OU have read in earlier pages how, when certain acts are performed over and over again, they become habits, and no conscious decision is necessary. You may not be aware of any mental process between your sensing the need to act, and the act itself. While you are talking to a friend, you become aware of a thread on your coat sleeve. Without thinking, you remove it. Your mind is spared the effort of making a conscious decision. Your conversation proceeds without interruption. Mere awareness of the thread is sufficient to bring about your action.

In the case of more important matters needing a decision, a definite effort of will is necessary. You must first form a mental image of what the results will be. The greater the degree to which you can direct your imagination and concentrate it upon this image, the greater the possibility that the decision will be a right one, and that it will be effectively carried out.

In the first chapter, you discovered how habit can be made to regulate your daily life ; how the development of good habits provides the background for smooth, well-regulated behaviour. All your normal, day to day comings and goings can be provided for by training your habits, then will-power is not needed for the performance of routine actions. Normally, you stand up, walk, talk, and eat, without effort of will, once you have formed the appropriate series of muscular habits.

WILL-POWER SHOULD NOT BE NEEDED IN LARGE QUANTITIES

In acting according to habit, the most important thing is the absence of conflicting emotions in your mind. Often, on a cold winter's morning, you have probably hesitated to get out of bed. In your imagination, you have felt the cold and, in contrast, you have reflected how warm the bedclothes are. You may even have lain for a long time trying to summon the will power to rise.

If you have made a habit of rising, regardless of whether it is freezing, and this habit has become deep seated in your mental make-up, then the effort required to rise will not be great.

Or, if you have disciplined yourself so that you are able to concentrate upon doing, and *not* dreaming about doing then, likewise, less effort will be required to translate thought into action. As soon as you can shut out from your mind the images of how cold it is likely to be, and how warm the bed is, your activity will cease to be suspended, and the way will be clear for your wish to get up to be expressed in a practical manner.

Thus, conflicting ideas prevent action : *action is only possible when conflict is removed.* The more you train yourself to shut out from your mind conflicting ideas, except the one to be expressed in activity, then the less mental energy, the less will-power, you will be called upon to exercise.

ORGANISE YOUR MIND, AND DEVELOP HEALTHINESS OF WILL

Healthiness of will is dependent upon self-control. Some mental images excite action more easily than others. Those connected with passions, appetites, emotions, feelings of pleasure, pain, or discomfort are very powerful. In comparison, ideals, courses of action to which you are unaccustomed, images not associated with pleasure, pain, or emotion, are less capable of moving you. The more ideal motives for behaviour must be strengthened by effort, if they are to find expression.

Where the will is to be healthy, it must be governed by knowledge ; subsequent action must follow the direction indicated by a knowledge of what is right, and not by feeling or emotion. Otherwise, unhealthiness of will is developed.

Untrained, uncontrolled anticipation of emotional pleasure may find active expression too quickly, before knowledge has been able to exercise restraint. Your self-control may be so weak that immediately the image of pleasurable experience comes into your mind, you must act to realise it, regardless of the consequences.

INTEREST THE SECRET OF WILL-POWER

Will-power depends to a tremendous extent on your deep and real interest; that is the heart of it. In its essence it is very simple. You are made in certain distinct ways and with definite instincts and abilities, and when you fulfil the purpose of your deepest nature, you find that you succeed with scarcely any thought of will-power at all.

The lesson to be learned from all this is that you should try to do the job in which you are truly interested. It has to be recognised that, in view of the fact that life is organised as it is, this is often far from easy. But it is possible to arouse interest in yourself on most subjects if you set out to do so. If you master a subject, you almost always do become interested in it to a certain extent.

A man may have wanted to teach and have known that he was especially fitted for that occupation. Unfortunately his parents perhaps could not provide the means for him to get the higher education that was necessary to achieve this ambition. So he may have drifted into something else and may know very well that his position is very far from being the ideal one.

WHEN INTEREST SEEMS LACKING

In this situation you may say that it will be difficult for the man to develop much will-power to work at his job. But the fact is that, with men under him or working with him, he has still the opportunity to teach others. And if he realises this fact and develops his interest on these lines his will-power for his work will automatically develop too.

The best way of managing life is to realise that you should not be forced to show excessive will-power in normal circumstances. If you do, it rather suggests you are, and have been, " driving the car with the hand-brake on." You ought to have sufficient interest in what you have to do for it to attract you so that you do it freely and happily.

Sometimes, of course, your interest is remote from the task in hand. And then you have to be stern with yourself. Many a man has wanted to be a doctor. He has known for certain that that profession is ideal for him. Yet some branches of the necessary study he has found very tiresome. Only by keeping in mind very clearly the final purpose for which he is working has he been able to master his desire to slack and instead been able to use will-power to carry on.

EXERCISES IN WILL-POWER FOR EVERY DAY

As a beginning, set yourself objectives that will present just a few difficulties. The following specific exercises will give point to your efforts, if you carry them out conscientiously.

1. Choose a book of a type you would normally consider dull and make yourself read one page of it every day. In order to prevent " skipping," make a summary of each page as you finish it. The important part of this exercise is to make yourself read the whole book.

2. Take a quarter of an hour's walk every day for a month, whatever the weather or however reluctant you feel. Take the walk at the same time each day and never for less than the time you decide upon.

THIS CHAPTER HAS TOLD YOU

1. Habit and imagination cannot alone deal with all situations. Will-power is often needed to carry through your decision.

2. Will-power should not be needed in large quantities. If it is, probably conflicting ideas are clogging the initiative of the person concerned.

3. Exclude any idea that conflicts with your objective. Accept the idea that means action. Then will-power will come automatically and easily.

4. Organise your self-control. Keep your impulses under control, and apply knowledge as a guide to action. Do not let the immediate emotion necessarily control you.

5. If you can arouse your own interest, will-power will come as a natural consequence.

6. Tenacity of purpose may be made into a strong habit. Do the will-power exercises on page 33.

4. IMPROVING CONCENTRATION AND ATTENTION

Every moment of your life, whether you are asleep or awake, things are happening around you ; the majority pass unnoticed ; a few are recorded in your mind, mostly temporarily, sometimes permanently. Have you ever paused to consider how far you really are aware of everything that is occurring ? Why do you become conscious of certain people, certain objects, and remain quite unconscious of others ?

The reason is that the capacity of your mind for absorbing impressions from the outside world is limited. If the greatest use is to be made of this capacity, it is important that you should select those items from your everyday life to which it will be most useful for you to devote your attention.

It is not always possible to do this. Certain experiences, by reason of their vividness, or intensity, force themselves into your field of attention, to the exclusion of everything else. Abnormally loud noises, bright colours, unusual occurrences, compel you to attend to them. But you can control your attention and concentrate it upon work which you are called upon to do, people and objects you are interested in, and want to know more about, and so on.

DISPERSED AND CONCENTRATED ATTENTION

You have probably known moments when your mind is a complete blank, when everything around you is a confused blur. Such a period is one of what is called dispersed attention. Then, suddenly, you rouse yourself; attention becomes concentrated upon a single object; life begins to move forward again.

The opposite of dispersed attention is concentrated attention, when your mind is so absorbed in the interest of the moment that you are oblivious to everything else. At tense moments during football matches spectators forget the discomfort of being in a crowd, the rain that may be falling, everything except the actions of the men on the field.

Another type of dispersed attention is seen when you attempt to attend to several things at once. For example, you may try to watch oncoming traffic while crossing a road, and, at the same time, observe two dogs fighting on the opposite pavement. Neither traffic nor dogs will receive your complete attention, with possibly unfortunate results.

A woman cannot concentrate effectively upon learning to knit, and also carry on a conversation. If she does, neither will be performed properly. But if one activity is reduced to a habit, then attention is free for the effective performance of other activities: the woman who has learnt to knit no longer finds it essential to concentrate upon each stitch.

VOLUNTARY AND INVOLUNTARY CONCEN-TRATION

The immature, undeveloped mind is at the mercy of everything intruding upon it. The child attends to the loudest noise, the brightest colour—any stimulus that has an exciting quality. Its attention drifts from one object to another.

The mature mind selects as the objects of attention those happenings which are related to permanent interests and purposes, and excludes all others.

To do this requires training—the cultivation of the habit of controlling the direction of attention, a rigorous exclusion of all irrelevant distractions from the field of consciousness. When you reach this stage, you become more the master of yourself, and less the slave of your environment. Your mind belongs to *you*, and not to every object that happens to catch your attention.

Voluntary attention requires effort, which will vary according to the interest you can find in the material upon which you desire to concentrate, and the intensity of other distractions. It is most difficult to concentrate upon things that have no meaning, or no relation to your needs and interests. Concentration is made easier if you discover meaning and interest in what you do. Your attention continually wanders from that which is meaningless. *Make a point of finding out the implications of everything you do, then the effort of attending will be diminished. Your task will be done better.*

GIVE YOURSELF BEST POSSIBLE PHYSICAL CONDITIONS

Voluntary attention becomes more difficult if your involuntary attention is being continually excited by your surroundings. Concentration upon a mathematical problem is difficult if someone is talking to you, if the wireless set is going, if a multitude of other excitements are clamouring for your attention. Writing a letter becomes an effort if your pen is scratching, or if the light is bad.

Give yourself a chance to concentrate. Do not handicap yourself by tolerating an environment full of minor and unnecessary distractions. Nearly always they can be removed without difficulty ; the scratching pen must be replaced, the bad light improved, the noise shut out, and so on.

Bodily states may impede concentration. A healthy body, free from ills and pains, is a valuable aid to controlled attention. So, too, is a mind which is kept clear of fears and inferiority feelings and all other such factors. Obviously it is very difficult to concentrate if some emotional conflict is dividing the mind.

Certain times of the day are also more favourable for concentration than others, though they do tend to vary for individuals. In general, the early morning is better than late at night, and it is a good plan, when possible, to get the most difficult tasks done before noon.

TRAINING ATTENTION BY OBSERVATION

Voluntary attention can be greatly strengthened by training yourself to observe accurately, for in order to observe you must pay attention. Possibly you think that very little escapes your notice, but tests show it is remarkable how little *is* noticed by most people. Police officers have the greatest difficulty in obtaining reliable descriptions of wanted persons. Can you say with assurance the colour of the eyes of men and women you meet daily ?

C. E. M. Joad once wrote in this connec-

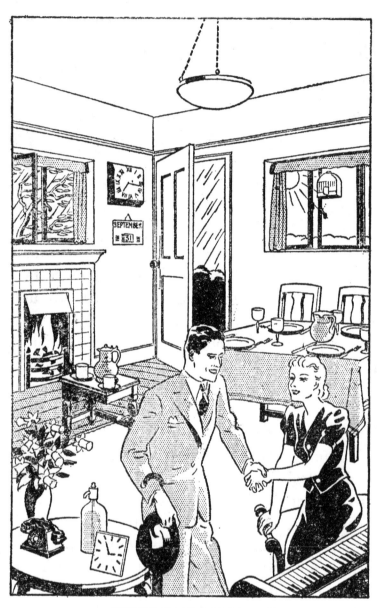

OBSERVATION TEST

There are twenty-two mistakes in this illustration. How many can you spot? The answer will be found on page 60

tion :—" At a Psychology Congress held at Göttingen, a clown suddenly burst into the Congress Hall closely pursued by a negro. The negro caught him, leapt upon him, and bore him to the floor, where a fight ensued, which was ended by a pistol shot, after which the clown got up and rushed out of the room, still closely pursued by the negro. The whole scene, which had been carefully rehearsed and photographed in advance, took less than twenty seconds. The President then informed the Congress that judicial proceedings might have to be taken, and asked each member to write a report, stating exactly what had occurred.

" Forty reports were sent in. Of these, one only contained less than twenty per cent of mistakes in regard to the principal facts : fourteen contained from twenty per cent. to forty per cent. mistakes ; thirteen contained more than fifty per cent. mistakes. In twenty-four, ten per cent. of the details recorded were pure inventions. In short, ten of the accounts were quite false, ranking as myths or legends, twenty-four were half legendary, and six only were even approximately exact."

If you have difficulty in training your attention on any subject you wish, give yourself practice in observation every day. Try and fix in your mind the order and nature of the shops in the main street nearest your home. Make a point of noticing the distinctive mannerisms of your friends. Set yourself to observe the colour of their eyes and hair, the shape of their hands and nails.

You will soon find your interest is aroused and your powers of attention will grow automatically. From time to time give yourself the following test.

Ask a friend to cover a small table with a number of miscellaneous objects—a penknife, cigarette case, reel of cotton, pair of gloves, etc. Look at the table for a given period of time, five minutes, ten minutes or a quarter of an hour. Then go away and write down everything you saw on the table. This will serve to test your observation and to train your memory at the same time.

EXERCISES IN EVERYDAY CONCENTRATION

Let us now consider how you might train yourself to attend to some daily routine task which you find difficulty in carrying out because your thoughts continually wander to other matters.

1. Discover an interest in your task, deriving this interest from whatever result is attached to it. If something you are called upon to do does not immediately awaken your attention because

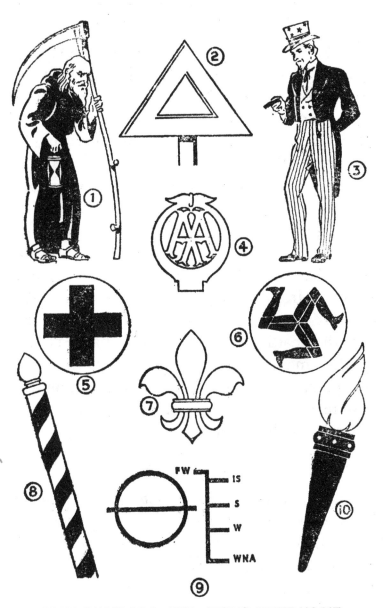

TEN SYMBOLS AND SIGNS EVERYONE
SHOULD KNOW

After you have tried to identify them turn to page 61

of its inherent interest, you must create an interest. Take the most boring part of your work, upon which, hitherto, you have found it difficult to concentrate ; strive to understand the significance of your duties, find meaning in them, and concentration will be made easier.

2. Here is another exercise in concentration. You may be troubled by an incapacity to absorb a difficult passage you are reading, or unable to concentrate upon complicated instructions. It will be easier to keep your attention from wandering if you re-echo the words in your mind. To-morrow, when you read the leading article in your daily paper, try this method, and discover how it helps you ignore other distractions ; the meaning will become more quickly apparent to you; concentration will be more easily possible.

THIS CHAPTER HAS TOLD YOU

1. Your attention is limited ; you can only know a certain amount about what is going on around you. Attention can be dispersed or concentrated.

2. Concentration can be voluntary or involuntary. It can be compelled from without, or it can be controlled from within and focused as desired.

3. Give yourself the best possible conditions for concentrating. Get rid of exterior distractions. Have quiet, the right light, etc.

4. Inability to concentrate may be due to internal distractions.

5. Certain times of the day are better for concentration than others. The morning is usually the best.

6. Observation exercises offer a good method of training the attention from which concentration springs. Use the concentration exercises on pages 42 and 44.

5. HOW TO IMPROVE YOUR MEMORY

PSYCHOLOGISTS define memory as the knowledge of experiences of which we have not been thinking with the additional awareness that we have experienced them before. The first essential in memory is to conjure up in the mind a picture of an event.

For instance, if you want to recollect who scored a certain goal in a football match, the first thing to do is to recall to your mind's eye the position of the field when the goal was scored. As you see the players in their places they will begin to move again as they did at the time and you will soon remember who made the winning shot.

A remarkable example of the power of mental pictures to assist memory is shown in the following story of Henri de Blowitz, the famous French journalist. He was present in a non-professional capacity, during an important speech of M. Thiers at Versailles. " When he had left," wrote de Blowitz, " a wild idea came into my head. Following an old idea which I still retain, I sat down and closed my eyes. I then strove to call up the image of the scene and, as I had listened very attentively to what he had said, it seemed as if I could hear him speaking and that I could write down his speech.

" I went at once to the telegraph-office in the Rue de Grenelle. I obtained writing materials in an empty room. There I put into operation my process for memorising. Alternately, I shut my eyes to see and hear M. Thiers, and then opened them to write out the speech for the wire. I was able to recall and report all his speech, which was, of course, instantaneously transmitted to London."

It is impossible to remember anything you have not experienced. Ease and vividness in recalling depends on the impression originally made upon your mental structure. An impression is unlikely to be made if you have not registered the experience in your mind by attending to it. The strength of the impression corresponds to the degree in which your mind is concentrated upon the particular event. If you are attending to other matters as well—that is, if your concentration is dispersed—the impression is weak, and capacity for revival is affected in proportion. Thus memory is the child of concentration.

THREE ASPECTS OF MEMORY TECHNIQUE

The three elements in memory are :

1. *Attention*, involving concentration upon

the experience to be registered in the mind.

2. *Retention,* or the process of mental registration, so that the experience may be recalled.

3. *Recall,* or recollection.

Let us consider the process of recall in more detail. How do we recollect? How do we train ourselves to recollect relevant experiences at the right time? How do we act in relation to events we know we must recall at definite times in the future?

In training your capacity for recollection at appropriate moments, you must form an association between the mental image of what is to be remembered, and another image or experience which you know will occur at the time when you wish recollection to take place.

For example, your wife asks you to bring home a bunch of flowers. You tie a piece of string around your little finger, so that you will not forget. You associate the idea of bringing home the flowers with the string on your finger. The string on your finger will be seen frequently during the day, and each time will recall the mental association between it and the flowers.

Recollection is thus dependent upon the

mental association of one event or object with others. The effectiveness with which you create these associations determines the effectiveness of your recollection.

FINER POINTS OF MEMORISING

Some minds are like jelly that yields to any pressure, but only with difficulty retains any impression permanently. Other minds are capable of retaining everything once experienced. Minds differ in natural retentiveness, both as between individuals, and in the same individual at various stages of his life. Recollection is correspondingly affected.

The man whose experiences, when he has selected them, stick in his mind, is the one who will progress. Others, whose minds either naturally, or through lack of training, are not so retentive, often spend a considerable part of their time relearning what they have forgotten.

If your mind is not naturally retentive, you must compensate for this disability by concentrating more upon connecting your selected experiences by association with your experience as a whole. The more you think over the experiences you wish to remember, the more they will become woven into associations with each other, and so the greater will be the ease with which one will recall the other.

Associations connected with your interests are the most easily formed. If you are interested in cricket, your ability to recollect dates in English history may be poor, but you will be able to retail to your friends the performances of outstanding players during the season. If your business interests are related to, say, wireless, you will be able to remember an extraordinary number of facts about the subject, owing to the amount of thinking you do about it. On the other hand, you may not be able to recall the name of a single racehorse, just because your interests do not lie in that direction.

THE WAY TO IMPROVE DIFFERENT ASPECTS OF YOUR MEMORY

Images or experiences recalled may be divided into the five types already described in our chapter on imagination :

1. *Visual* (by sight).
2. *Tactile* (by touch).
3. *Auditory* or *Oral* (by hearing).
4. *Odile* (by smell).
5. *Muscular*.

One type of image frequently recalls another. You may associate specific scents with certain flowers ; the sight of a hyacinth may recall to you a mental image of one odour, jasmine, another. When you pass the Albert Hall, you may recollect music you have heard at a concert.

The more of these combinations or associations you form in your mind in connection with an experience, the more permanent will be your capacity for recollecting it. If you register in your mind what anything looks, feels, sounds, and smells like, you will be able to recall it more easily than if you only register what it looks like.

USING ALL YOUR SENSES

Suppose, for example, on your last summer holiday, your mind was impressed by the warmth of the sun, the touch of the water on your skin, the smell of the sea, the sounds of children playing on the sands and your pleasurable sensations when swimming and walking. Six months later, any chance reminder to any one of these senses—touch, smell, hearing—will evoke the whole scene before you. If you only registered what the place looked like, you are much less likely to remember it afterwards.

The wisest and most effective way of improving your memory is by developing your habitual method of registering facts in your mind. Repetition is the most commonly employed procedure. You learn poetry by repeating it over and over to yourself.

Another, is by intensifying the experience so that attention must be concentrated upon it. Sometimes, in books, items which it is important you should remember may be underlined, printed in larger letters, or heavier type. These may be described as the mechanical methods of memorising.

In addition to the purely mechanical methods of memorising, the systematic method is that which attaches meaning to experiences, analysing and classifying them into systems. Words which have a meaning for you, are more easily remembered than those which have none. If you form words into sentences, make sentences have a rhythmic association with each other, as in poetry, they are easier to memorise than if such associations are not created.

FACES AND NAMES

It has probably happened that you have met a person and been introduced to him but, when you met him again, while you recognised his face, you could not recall his name. The reason is that you have failed to form in your mind an association between the visual image of what he looks like, and the oral image of his name, so that one spontaneously recalls the other.

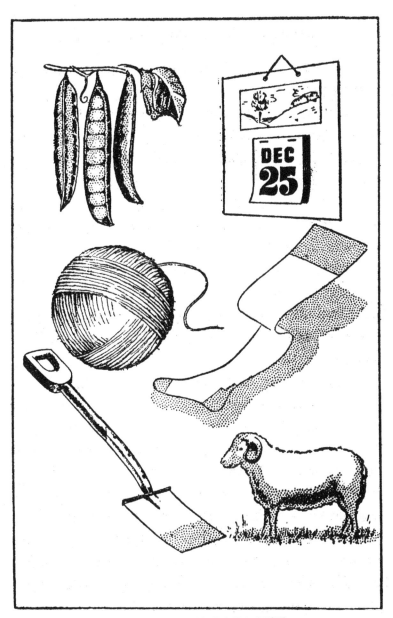

A MEMORY EXERCISE

Since it is established that the easiest way to remember a number of varied objects is to find some associating link, what is the best way of remembering the six items illustrated? The answer
is on page 61

You can strengthen the associative link at the time when the introduction is made, by concentrating upon forming as many associations as possible between his name, the oral image, and his facial characteristics, or the visual image.

For example, he may be introduced to you as Mr. Brown. He may have brown eyes, brown hair, brown skin. Associate these characteristics with his name. Then, when you see him again, visual and oral images will be recalled simultaneously. Other names may not be so easy. Nevertheless, associations should be possible.

Suppose you are introduced to a Mr. Blenkinsop. His name starts with Bl. You note that he has blue eyes. Blue also starts with the letters Bl. Once you have formed this association, it will be easier to associate your image of his face with his name. In other words, whenever you wish to register in your mind two images so that they will be recalled together in the future, concentrate upon finding a common link that will associate them—inseparably tie them together. One cannot, of course, give a formula for remembering every single surname. The point is that one should *whenever possible* strengthen the associative link by such simple means as have just been indicated.

In trying to recall, you should always give yourself a fair chance. Remember you will do better when feeling confident and in good health than when you are depressed or tired. So, if you have to make a special effort of memory, see that you are in good condition for it.

COAXING YOUR MIND TO REMEMBER

At the same time, there are various other ways in which you can coax your mind to work. A modern psychologist has written :

" Look squarely at the person whose name you wish to recall, avoid doubts as to your ability to recall it ; for doubt is itself a distraction. Put yourself back into the time when you formerly used this person's name."

Sometimes you find it is not easy to recall what you feel you ought to know perfectly well. It is on the " tip of your tongue " but you cannot quite recall it. The correct method at such a time is not to hurry the mind, but to wait for a minute or two. Such a pause often helps to recall what you want to know in a way that active search does not.

There are a number of hindrances to recall. Emotional disturbances check it. Fear especially can do this. You see this particularly in stage fright. Many a speaker with a splendid outline of his speech and a number of clever epigrams in mind, finds that fright obliterates these, and he has to sit down knowing that the best parts of his speech have been left unspoken.

The only effective remedy against such a difficulty is knowledge of how to keep your emotions in check so that they do not swamp your mind. It is true that many systems have been devised to help memorising and in some cases, and to a certain extent, they are undoubtedly useful. But it has been said that whoever relies upon a complicated memory-system resembles a tight-rope walker so intent upon keeping his equilibrium as to be unable to attend to anything else.

WHEN TO FORGET

The capacity of your mind to store up images and the associations between them is limited. You cannot register everything so that you can hope to recall it, any more than you can attend to everything that is happening around you. If you consciously endeavour to remember too much, you will defeat your own object, and remember nothing.

The late Sir Arthur Conan Doyle once made his hero, Sherlock Holmes, give expression to a

very significant statement. It was to the effect
that the great detective of fiction sought to
memorise only those items of experience per-
tinent to his purpose, and then only to a
limited extent. With regard to everything else,
all he sought to do was to memorise where the
relevant information might be obtained.

Compared with the sum total of knowledge,
only a very limited amount can be woven into
the structure of your memory. But you can
memorise where the other knowledge is avail-
able—in libraries, from other people, and so
on. So far as everyday facts are concerned, you
can afford to forget many of them ; you *must*,
if your mind is not to be overburdened with
detail. At the same time, however, you must
keep a mental reference file, so to speak, which
will enable you to know at once where you can
secure information if the need for it should arise.

SPEEDS OF MEMORISING

Ability to memorise is partly inborn, as we
have seen. Some fortunate persons have only
to read over a passage once, see a picture for a
moment, and the details are indelibly imprinted
upon their memory. Others must read the
passage many times, or concentrate for a long
period upon a picture, before their minds will
record it with any degree of precision.

If you belong to the latter type, you can, to some extent, compensate for your disability, and increase your speed of memorising, by reading meaning into what you are memorising, developing a rich association structure about it, systematising it. Or, if you are fortunate to possess a naturally good capacity for memorising, you can improve your speed of memorising still more by following the same procedure.

EXERCISES TO "POLISH UP YOUR MEMORISING"

1. As a beginning in training your memory, take a picture in your daily paper. Study it for half a minute. Then put it to one side. Recall and write down what you have seen. You will find that the more meaning you have been able to read into the picture, the more complete will be your ability to recall every detail.

2. Take a paragraph of printed matter. Slowly read it over once. Then try to write it out. Again, the more you have been able to systematise the material, and give it meaning, the more you will remember.

3. Take a short poem which appeals to you and read it over carefully three or four times, making sure you have grasped the succession of ideas and pictures it presents. Then put

the book away and see how much of the poem you can repeat. In doing this exercise you are advised to learn the whole poem at one time. Experiments have shown it is easier to grasp and retain a complete sequence of thought, than to remember isolated lines or phrases in their correct order. If you grasp the meaning it will be easier to remember the words which express the meaning.

4. Finally, if your memory does not improve as rapidly as you would like, or if it is a constant source of weakness, make a properly kept diary and appointments pad do its work for you. You must be rigidly systematic in this matter. Enter every appointment as it is made ; list your duties every day and cross off each one as it is fulfilled ; note down telephone numbers, addresses, etc., *in their proper place*, as soon as you learn them.

THIS CHAPTER HAS TOLD YOU

1. Memory can only be good if the original occasion called forth concentration. Shutting your eyes and visualising a scene will often bring it all back to you.

2. Memory's three main aspects are attention, retention and recall. Recollection depends upon associating one object or event with others.

3. Powers of memorising differ. But a person with a

poor memory can make up for this by memory training. Link your interests with what you have to memorise.

4. *Memory works through sight, sound, smell and touch. These are the visual, auditory, odile and tactile faculties. Each helps the others in memorising.*

5. *Faces and names can be remembered by forming mental associations. Sometimes the mind needs to be coaxed rather than bullied into remembering.*

6. *It is possible to improve your speed of memorising. Memory exercises are on page 58.*

ANSWERS TO ILLUSTRATION TESTS

Page 40. The mistakes in the picture are : (1) There is no hearth in front of the fire. (2) The man and the girl are shaking hands with their left hands. (3) The black piano keys should be in groups of two and three, not two and four. (4) There is a window where the chimney should be. (5) The two clocks show different times. (6) There is no numeral VIII on the big clock and the two VII's are inverted. (7) The man's coat is buttoned right over left. (8) The girl's coat is buttoned left over right. (9) The door knob is in the wrong place. (10) One of the lamp chains is missing. (11) The daffodils have the wrong leaves. (12) One leg of the stool is missing. (13) The calendar shows the impossible date of September 31st. (14) The sun is shining through the window, while rain can be seen through the door. (15) The bird-cage is not connected with the ceiling by any means. (16) The soda syphon has no lever. (17) The knives and forks are on the wrong sides of each plate. (18) The lip of the water-jug is in the wrong place. (19) Two of the wine glasses have no base. (20) On the telephone dial the holes for numbers should not continue round in a complete circle. In actual fact only ten holes should be shown. (21) There is no cord to the telephone receiver. (22) The wind is blowing the tree one way, but the rain is being blown in the opposite direction.

Page 43.   The ten illustrations are : (1) " Father Time." (2) Danger sign. (3) " Uncle Sam " (America). (4) Automobile Association Badge. (5) Red Cross—Ambulance or Hospital sign. (6) Isle of Man coat of arms. (7) The Boy Scout Badge. (8) A barber's pole. (9) Plimsoll line loading mark on ships. (10) Traffic sign for a school.

Page 53.   The easiest way to get some connection between the objects, is this : December 25 (Christmas), Stocking (Darning), Ball of Wool (Where does it come from ?), Sheep (lamb), Green Peas (Gardening), Spade.

WHAT THE NEXT BOOK TELLS YOU

WHAT can stop our progress when we have brought mental efficiency to a reasonable working level ?

In average circumstances, nothing. But there is one trouble which many of even the cleverest of people meet at times.

It has been called the plague of the twentieth century. And it has the vague and all-embracing name of " nerves." To most people, nerves may mean anything from a headache or a slight attack of indecision, to the other extreme of a complete breakdown.

This is the subject of Book 5 which you will be reading next, under the title of " HOW TO CONTROL YOUR NERVES."

You will learn how to adjust your life to the stresses and strains of modern living, and how to combat that overwrought feeling.

You will learn how to keep healthy, happy and efficient, despite the " plague of the twentieth century."

Printed in Great Britain

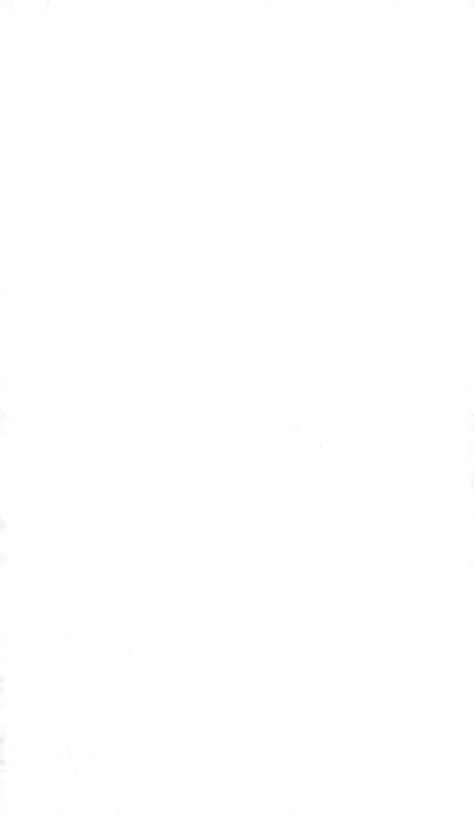

Printed in the USA
CPSIA information can be obtained
at www.ICGtesting.com
LVHW020030100224
771465LV00011B/188